# KUNG FU FOR GIRLS

## Self-Defense with Style

# KUNG FU FOR GIRLS

## Self-Defense with Style

### By Simon Harrison

Library of Congress Cataloging in Publication Number: 2003113710

ISBN 1-931686-93-9

First published in Great Britain in 2003
Printed in China

Typeset in Chalet Comprime and Myriad Condensed

Designed by Andrea Stephany

Distributed in North America by Chronicle Books
85 Second Street
San Francisco, CA 94105

10 9 8 7 6 5 4 3 2 1

First published by
Ebury Press
Random House
20 Vauxhall Bridge Road, London SW1V 2SA

Quirk Books
215 Church Street
Philadelphia, PA 19106

# Acknowledgments

Dedicated to Mum, Dad, and the rest of the family.

Thanks to Philip King for knowing a good idea when he sees one, very special thanks to the lovely Njong and Yasmine, 3 is the magic number, cheers mad Dave. Thanks to A.M.A. & Co.

**!**

When attempting the exercises and/or advice given in this book, you should proceed with due care and caution. The exercises and suggestions are guidelines for a healthy individual, and if you have any medical condition or are unsure whether you should perform certain exercises, please consult your doctor. The Publisher and Author cannot accept responsibility for illness, injury, damage, or economic loss due to the use or misuse of the information and advice contained in this book.

# Contents

**Introduction** 8

**Basics** 10

**Tools** 28

**Techniques** 50

**Moves** 66

**Index** 111

# Introduction

*Kung Fu for Girls* can be your pocket bodyguard. Carry it around with you, and it will help you take care of yourself wherever you are. In *Kung Fu for Girls* you will find simple and practical self-defense techniques. Practice them with friends before you go out in the evening. They can be fun—and if you do them properly they will keep you safe from harm.

Simplicity is vital to successful self-defense. Your motto from now on is "Keep It Simple. Simple Is Effective." The initial letters spell KISSIE so, to help commit your objectives to memory, you should be saying KISSIE KISSIE to yourself over and over.

Your personal attitude to yourself and your surroundings is your first and most important barrier against the street criminal. Self-defense is also about stopping trouble before it starts. Knowing a few simple moves will increase your confidence; you'd be surprised how many potential attackers may well detect this and end up looking for an easier target.

A helpful motto for when you perceive a dangerous situation is "Turn Around and Run Away" or TA-RA for short. This is usually very effective, but if running away isn't an option, use some of the techniques from this book. Be creative—whether you use your favorite kitten heels or a cell phone, use them to full effect and walk away unharmed. The sense of satisfaction will be immense.

You never know, you might even get a taste for kung fu. If so, I suggest you build on what you've learned here by attending professional classes.

So now, get ready to enter a whole new world of kung fu—for women.

*Simon Harrison*

Note: The directions and techniques that follow generally assume that you are right-handed. Swap them if you are left-handed.

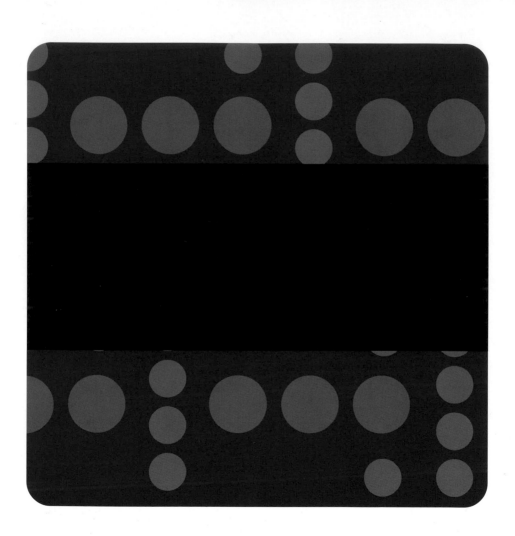

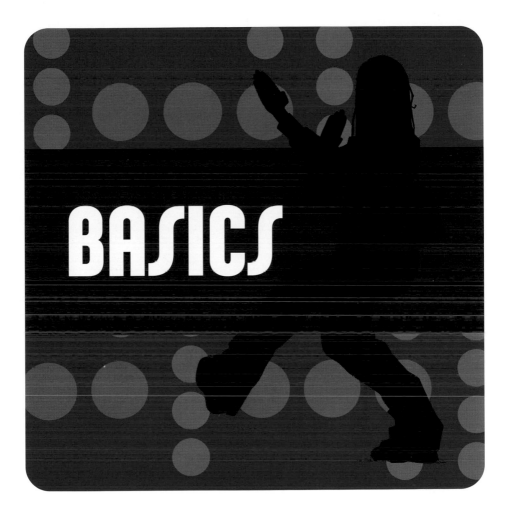

# Attitude

Imagine four women. They all look like you. One is casually dressed, confident. The second, a lost tourist. Next comes a nervous one in heels and a long coat. The last is also casually dressed but talking into a cell phone. Now imagine you are a misogynistic street crook. Which one of the "yous" would you target first? List them in order of priority. There are a few key characteristics that make you vulnerable to attack:

 Showing fear or being overtly nervous.

 Looking lost, wearing restrictive clothing.

 Not paying attention and displaying expensive treats such as minidisk players and cell phones.

# Awareness and Antisurveillance

Cultivate a preventive attitude.

The catchphrase for the street is "be prepared and be aware." Like it or not, the street is a hostile environment. If you are the sort of person who never worries about being attacked and keeps an eye on her surroundings, you will probably never have a problem. But if you are anxious, here are a few tips.

Be aware of transitional phases. It takes the mind a few moments to adjust between one environment and another; for example, the transition from escalator to subway exit. You are still digesting the information from the interior environment as you exit, which can make you vulnerable and careless. Before you leave, take a look around. (The same applies to transitions from a bus, restaurant, office, or even your home.) Looking around is an act of antisurveillance: it's a simple precaution that can put off a criminal because he sees you are aware and therefore not soft. You become a potential hazard—unpredictable and therefore a non-target.

# Practice

Practice is essential. There is no substitute for practice and the perfection of movement you will accomplish by repeating the techniques with a partner. (Except maybe dumb luck, which you simply can't rely on.) The point of practice is to create what is called "muscle memory." When you learned to walk or to catch a ball, you created muscle memory. The idea with kung fu is to create muscle memory that is so efficient it bypasses the conventional avenues of physical behavior, deeply embedding complex reactions to dangerous situations in your nervous system. Good kung fu is mindless. It's an expression of your body with minimum interference from the intellect. It's how animals react.

# Stance

How you stand is of fundamental importance. I am not talking about the flashy pose you strike. I'm referring to how strongly you are attached to the ground. Terms like "steady," "well-grounded," and "rooted" are appropriate here. The stronger your stance, the harder you will be able to hit your attacker. It's a simple principle. If you are immovable and you hit someone, he moves, but you don't.

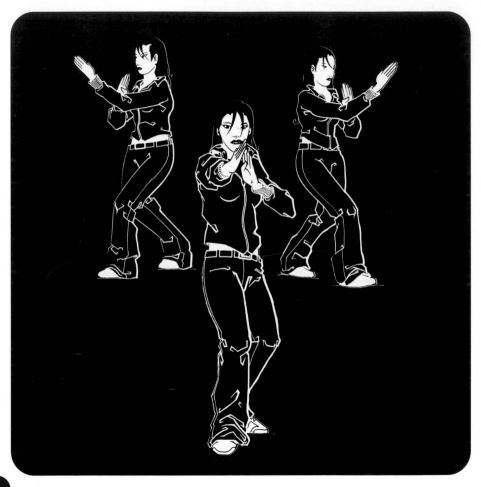

# Guard Positions

Here we have a left-handed and right-handed guard position. Study the front view carefully. It's arranged so that the hands can protect the face or body very quickly. They guard the center line of your body. The knees are bent, balanced, and ready to kick or spring in any direction. In combat you move on the balls of your feet. Flat-footed stances are stronger, but you need lots of practice to use them effectively.

This is just one of many guard positions.

# The Center Line

Attacking criminals are attracted to your center line like insects to lamplight. They will direct their attacks almost exclusively to this region. They seek to undermine your balance and composure on every level. They attack your "heart"—the very core of your being. Sexual predators are particularly drawn to this region.

Put it this way: If your center line is an intimate dinner party for a few special friends, then the criminal street attacker is the gatecrasher from hell.

Guard your center line. And attack his. Your limbs are excellent protectors of your center line, as they can be used to kick, jab, gouge, scratch, elbow, knee, bite, and head-butt. Always come back to your center line when not engaged in grabbing, blocking, or attacking. It's a good habit.

Finally, don't just fall into a fighting stance at the drop of a hat. You'll ruin the surprise for the attacker when you start to slap him silly, and that wouldn't be fair. Maintain the element of surprise until the last possible instant.

Use any means at your disposal to win. Fight back and make him regret his decision to pick on you as a target. If your fighting is precise, measured, and accurate, he will stand little chance. You will walk away unharmed and a little wiser. That's good enough for me.

# Targets

Here is the dangerous thug. Great waves of greed and desire slosh about inside his head, overpowering all sense of reason and human dignity. He is a menace. But as he hurtles toward you, he suffers two major disadvantages. By assuming you are weak and therefore an easy target, he increases your element of surprise, making it a cinch for you to deck him. This guy is also oblivious to the fact that he is literally oozing weak points. Here are a few:

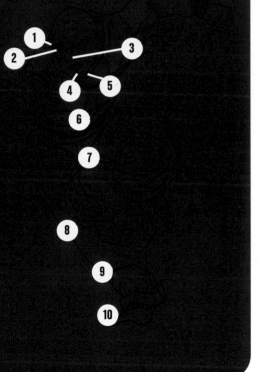

### 1 THE EARS.
Bite or grab them. Use them to manipulate his head. Slap them hard to deafen him.

### 2 THE EYES.
Jab and gouge them with your fingers. If he can't see you, he can't fight. Also, if you get the chance, spit in them.

### 3 THE NOSE.
Hit it with open palm strikes to cause watery eyes, to break the delicate bones, and to destroy his balance. His head will automatically tip back when hit on the tip of the nose. Just shove him onto his back. Grab the nostrils—they're great for moving his head around.

### 4 THE CHIN.
Hit it upward from below with elbows, palms, knees, or your head. Catch him while he's talking and he will bite his own tongue off. Also good for throwing him off balance.

### 5 THE THROAT AND NECK.
Strangle, gouge, and hit these areas. Nothing drops a man like a crushed larynx. Dig your fingers into the recess at the base of the throat between the collarbones.

### 6 THE BODY.
For more advanced students, aim at the body. Targets are the sternum, collarbones, solar plexus, ribs, and stomach. From behind, hit the spine, lower back, and nape of the neck.

### 7 THE GROIN.
Kick him in the gonads. Grab, knee, or, if necessary, bite. All are very effective.

### 8 THE KNEES.
Kick his knees with your feet to force them back the wrong way.

### 9 THE SHINS.
Scrape them with the edge of your shoe. (It takes the skin off.)

### 10 THE FEET.
Aim for the toes and the small delicate bones on the top of the foot.

# Blocks

### INSIDE BLOCK TO THE SIDE OF THE HEAD

Assume the guard position. With your front arm, perform a pseudo-military salute. Now move the saluting hand six inches forward, away from your head. Execute the movement again but go immediately to the finishing position illustrated. Any attack to the side of the head can be absorbed on the forearm. Your arm hacks into your attacker's like an ax hitting a tree branch.

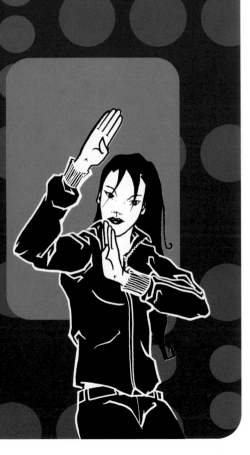

## DOUBLE-HANDED BLOCK

This block serves the same purpose as the inside block but is more heavily reinforced to absorb very powerful attacks. From the guard position, raise your hands to the side as if holding onto the dangling handle on a subway. That's the blocking posture. Attacks are absorbed on the outside edge of the forearms.

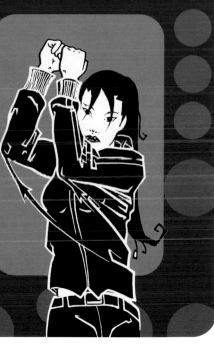

## LIFTING BLOCK

From the guard position, lift your forward arm and brush your hair back away from your forehead. Now imitate the same move again, but don't actually touch your head. This block will absorb an attack to the side of the head or a direct attack on the face if you catch it early enough.

## CIRCLING OUTER BLOCK

Hold up your hand in front of your face and imagine you are polishing a window. Circle your hand rapidly away from your body and then back to the point of origin. Attack impact is absorbed on the outer forearm.

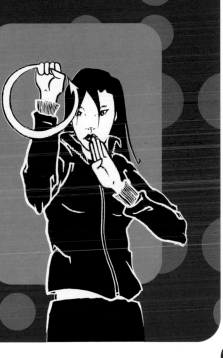

## CIRCLING INNER BLOCK

Exactly the same principle as the circling outer block, but you reverse the circle and block with the inner forearm.

## LOW WINDSHIELD-WIPER BLOCK

From the guard position, sweep your arm down in a hacking arc like the windshield-wiper of a car. This will block an attack to your body. Impact is absorbed on the outer forearm.

## THE SLAP BLOCK

Simply use the hook palm strike (page 43) to drive your attacker's arm off to the side. Contact is made with the palm. Don't use the fingers—they'll get bent backward and broken. Grabbing the sleeve of the aggressor makes it easier to control him.

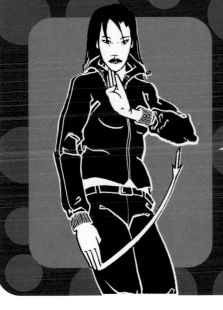

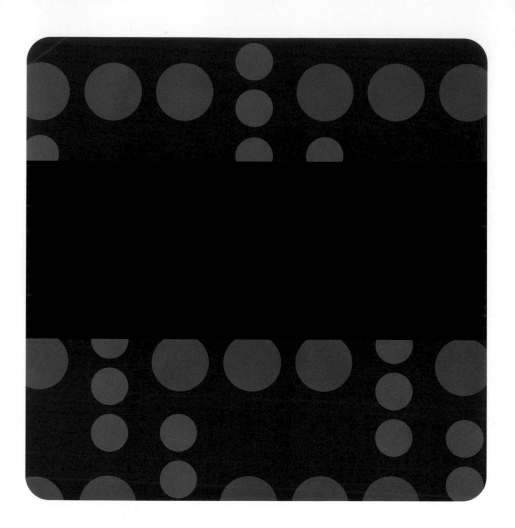

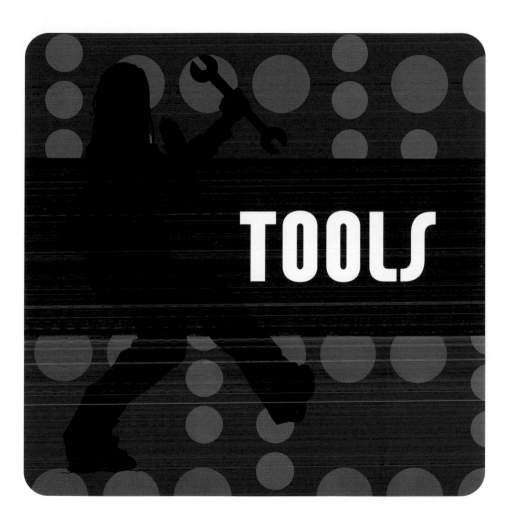

TOOLS

# Tools

**1 THE HANDS.**

Very versatile defense tools. Use fingertips to jab at the eyes and throat. Use nails to claw, gouge, and tear skin and eyes. The outside edge of the hand can chop at the larynx and nose. The back of the hand can be slapped across the target's nose and mouth. The palm of the hand can be used to slap, thrust, or push, and the knuckles can be used to punch, but try to avoid this as you may incur injuries.

**2 THE FOREARMS.**

Use the inside and outside edges to slam your attacker in the head or neck.

### 3 THE ELBOWS.

Deadly. Probably the hardest self-defense instrument on your upper body. It gets knocked about and leaned on so often that even the softest person has a conditioned, hard elbow. Use to jab and bludgeon.

### 4 THE SHOULDERS.

Good for knocking a man over when you have him off balance. Aim for the chest or abdomen.

### 5 THE HEAD.

This is a tricky tool because your head is a delicate area. The skull protects the brain so it must be hard; it can be used to butt the attacker's face, but if you're not used to the idea of doing this it can be quite a shock to the system. Be careful. It would be pointless to head-butt a man without the correct amount of conviction and succeed only in knocking yourself out. If you must butt, use your forehead. Try to avoid hitting him with your face, or you risk injuring yourself. (That would be grotesque—I've seen it happen.) If you're grabbed from behind, you can also use the back of your head—but, I say again, be careful.

### 6 THE BUTT.

Yes, your ass is a weapon. It can be used to hit and strike, as you will learn later (page 78).

### 7 THE KNEES.

Very strong. Probably the strongest weapon on your lower body, for reasons similar to those for the elbow. Knees have lots of leverage and make excellent close-quarter weapons. Be careful not to hit with your kneecap, though. Use the area starting just above the kneecap to about a third of the way up your thigh.

### 8 THE FEET.

They are tough, get stood on all day, and are usually covered in shoes, so make use of them. Use the heel, the ball of the foot, the top of the foot, the toes (if you are wearing rigid shoes), and the edges of the sole (for scraping bones).

## Give Him the Elbow

A lot of energy can be focused into your elbow. Leverage exerted from the waist is transmitted directly to the shoulder and loses little impetus before reaching the elbow. You actually hit with your waist, but the arms transmit the power. This is called technical strength. It's why a 125-pound woman can flatten a 180-pound man. To find the correct elbow position, imitate a chicken. Flap your stubby wings. Stop flapping and rotate at the waist.

Your elbows will create a slashing horizontal arc around your body. You simply swing and hit an attacker across the head, as illustrated.

The upward elbow strike is a vertical slashing motion of the elbow. Smell your armpit. Lift your arm and have a good sniff. This attack connects with the underside of the chin. The free hand keeps his arm at bay.

Now grab his arm and drag it down. If the opportunity arises and you find yourself with a height advantage over your attacker, you can use the downward elbow strike. The technique begins at the upward elbow position. It descends rapidly into your attacker's exposed neck or back.

High kicks look great on TV, but in a desperate fight they can be slow and too elaborate. A kick to the head is harder to effectively pull off than a stomp to the knee. Remember, "Keep It Simple. Simple Is Effective."

# Kicks

## THE FRONT GROIN KICK

From the guard position (page 17), raise your rear leg as if you are about to climb some steps. Then in one fluid motion, snap your leg straight. Keep the toes pointed and hit with the top of the foot and lower shin. After snapping the leg out, pull it back immediately like a twanged rubber band and put it down. Remain balanced throughout the whole procedure.

## GROIN KICK IN ACTION

It's the atomic bomb of the kick world, not because of its power but because of where it lands. Kick a man's groin and he will drop like a stone. It takes a hard man—no, let me rephrase that—it takes a eunuch or a monk to withstand a kick in the gonads. The beauty of this target is it's really hard to miss. Just aim between his knees—your foot will ricochet off the insides of his thighs like a pinball until it reaches the top. Then, exert some force!

## SIDE STOMP KICK

This is a very powerful kick. Lift the leg as illustrated. Thrust down and strike with the heel. Avoid hitting with the toes. They can bend back and get injured. Your leg is in a direct line with your body so that your weight is behind the kick, focused at the heel. The technique holds a lot of power, and is a good long-range defense against a knife attack.

## THE DOG LIFTS ITS LEG

Imitate a male dog lifting his leg to a fire hydrant. Place your foot on the knee of your attacker and thrust your leg straight to force his knee back the wrong way. The reflex reaction to this attack is to jerk to a halt, as men don't usually like having their knees broken. This movement can stop a man in his tracks.

### CROSS-STOMP KICK

This kick works best when snapped out like the other kicks. Pretend you're doing a Tae-Bo workout video. Just point your toes out and—boom! Hit with the heel. This can also be used to grind down a shin bone.

## GIVE HIM THE BOOT

A knee strike to the groin is a man's nightmare, but other body targets are also effective. Here, the attacker is pulled onto the blow, which doubles in power as it rises up to meet his falling body. Lift your leg high as if climbing steep steps. This is a fast, simple, close-quarter movement.

# Palm Strikes

You've all seen lengthy fistfights on TV. No one gets cut, knuckles don't even bleed. To know what it really feels like to punch someone's skull, try this quick test. Approach your bedroom door and punch it as hard as you can. Knuckles need to be properly aligned with forearm bones or you will sprain your wrist when you hit your target. Energy will dissipate into the wrist joint instead of up the forearm. Don't risk injury by punching people in fights—use palm strikes instead.

## THE HOOK PALM STRIKE

Palm striking is easy. From the guard position (page 17), thrust forward with either hand. Stretch back the fingers so the heel of the palm is exposed. This lowers the minimal risk of injury even further. You can curl your fingers as illustrated (below right, inset), if you prefer. You'll exert the same force, but some find it more comfortable.

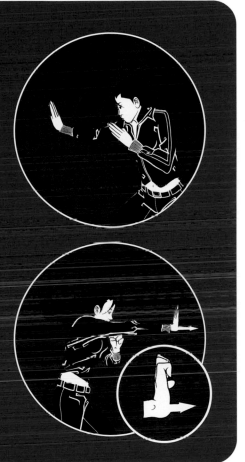

## GIVE HIM FIVE

Assume the guard position (page 17) and then imagine you're holding a beach ball directly in front of your face. The fingers point straight up. Pull one hand back and rotate your hips in that direction. The extended arm will form a slashing arc in front of your body, with the palm heel focusing the power. Thrust with hips and arm. Bash him on the jaw or ear.

## WEAPONS IN YOUR HANDBAG

**1 THE CELL PHONE.**
For use, see page 93.

**2 KEYS.**
Grip them so that they protrude from the bottom of your fist or so they protrude through the gaps between your knuckles to form a spiky fist. Use to jab, scratch, and gouge.

**3 COMBS.**
Use the same way you'd use keys (above) or a cell phone (page 93).

**4 LIPSTICK, MASCARA.**
Any longish, tough, plastic-packed accessory can be used to stab at your attacker's eyes and throat.

**5 A HANDFUL OF CHANGE.**
Hurl into the face of an attacker with a knife. This will give you time to escape. Quarters are the best, having a good size-to-weight ratio. But this can get expensive, so try not to meet too many rapists, muggers, or murderers on one journey!

**6 THE HANDBAG.**
Your purse itself can be used as a shield. The edges can be used to scuff at your attacker's face. You can use it to slap at his hands if he's holding a weapon.

# Stiletto Kung Fu: 1

High heels look great, but let's face it, they seem difficult to walk in comfortably and are nearly impossible to run in with any degree of safety. If you do have to fight in them, however, you might as well learn how to do it effectively. The heel can be used to stab at the attacker's feet, shins, knees, thigh muscles, groin, stomach, and ribs.

The point of the heel inflicts horrible pain because all the power of your kick is focused behind that little point. If your attacker is knocked down, use the heel to stomp on him so that he can't get up and chase you when you run away. Go for the ankles, knees, or hands.

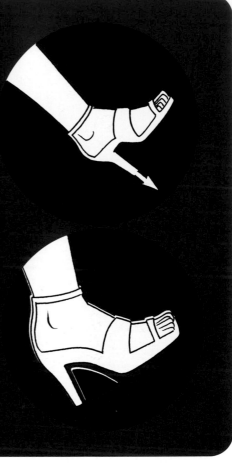

The inverted "V" of the heel (the empty area between the heel and the flat portion of the sole) is great for trapping limbs. It can easily grab the backs of knees (as illustrated below right). Simply turn the foot to the side using a side stomp (page 38) or a cross-stomp kick (page 40) to pin the limb from behind. This method is also great for grinding down the front of the shin bone.

# Stiletto Kung Fu: 2

If you are ever forced into a situation where you have to run for your life while wearing inappropriate footwear, try to take off your shoes. You must use your common sense here: You can't expect an attacker to pause while you fiddle with your shoe straps. Evaluate the situation and act accordingly. If you do get the high heels off, don't throw them away. Hold them as shown (facing page) and use them like ice picks to climb the craggy body and pitted face of any mugger stupid enough to stand in your way. Pay particular attention to the bony areas of the head and face. Shoes used in this way can cause shocking pain, and if you hit him hard in the head they can penetrate to the bone. He

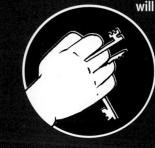

will drop like he's been shot through the head, so be careful when you use them. If you can't get your shoes off, use your keys—they're just as effective. Hold as shown at left. Stab downward at the head, neck, and body, or punch at the same targets.

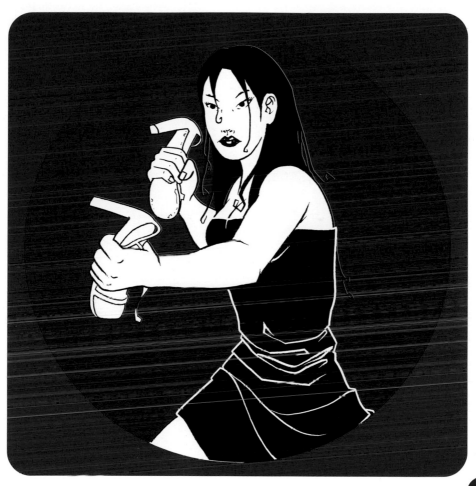

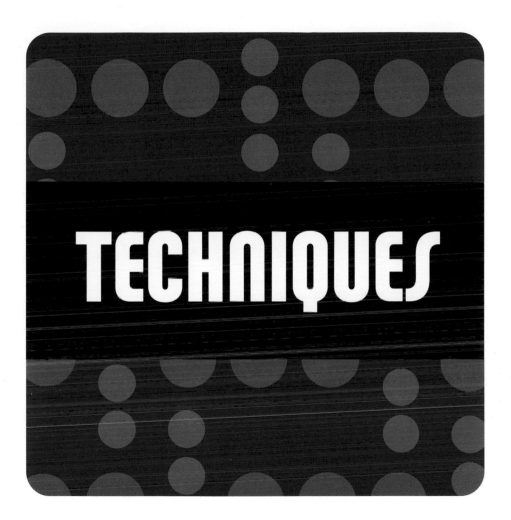

TECHNIQUES

The following pages are designed for you to see how techniques can be strung together to create combinations that flow in a logical sequence. Each move is dependent on your attacker's actions and his reactions to yours. The idea is to use your orientation and natural momentum to maximize the power of your counter-attacks and to manipulate your opponent so he is kept physically and psychologically off balance. This minimizes the chance of him hitting you again once you have blocked his initial attack.

These are highly confrontational counter-attacks, based on the assumption that you do not, as yet, have the necessary experience to step strategically, which is very hard to do properly and very easy to forget under pressure. Some strategic footwork maneuvers are included at the end of this section, and they are repeated later. If you can master the procedure and remember to use it when someone is trying to choke you, you will be practically street-invincible. In the meantime, here is how to deal with someone who is completely in your face.

# Technique 1

## BLOCK ...

The attacker swings a big drunken punch at the side of your head. Use a lifting, outer-circling, or double-handed block to dissipate the blow. You must counter-attack immediately.

**. . . GIVE HIM THE ELBOW . . .**
Grab his arm with the blocking hand and pull down to drag him off balance, then mash him across the jaw with a forward horizontal elbow strike. Watch out for flying teeth.

### ...GIVE HIM FIVE.

Let go of his arm and hit him with a hook palm strike to the face. He will be falling into the blow, so you may need to dance out of the way a bit and change your footing. Be prepared.

# Technique 2

## BLOCK . . .

This time, he reaches out to engulf your head with both arms and tries to wrestle you into a head-lock. Work your arms between his and push his elbows out.

## . . . GIVE HIM THE FINGER . . .

As soon as you get the opportunity, spread your fingers like a fan and dig them straight into his eyes. His attempted bear-hug is now obstructed by your arms, which are attacking him (and defending you). His head will tip back as you hit his eyes.

## ...GIVE HIM FIVE.

As he tips his head back, smack him hard on the chin. Use an open palm strike to destroy what little balance he has left and knock him flat on his back. Now would be a good time to follow up with a groin kick.

# Technique 3

**BLOCK . . .**

Block a direct punch to the face—or a grab for the throat—using lifting or outer-circling blocks.

## ...GIVE HIM THE ELBOW...

Pivot your whole body while simultaneously assuming the chicken wing strike posture, and slam the point of your elbow straight onto his nose. He will feel as if you stuck a 200-volt cable up his nostrils.

## ...GIVE HIM THE BOOT.

Rotate back the opposite way and catch him on the rebound. Grab the back of his neck or head and drag him down for a knee strike to the body, neck, or face. If you jerk his neck down fast enough, you can glve him whiplash to add to his troubles.

# Technique 4

### SIDE STEP 45 . . .

Step toward your attacker at 45 degrees. Cut across him as he lunges, making him overshoot and leaving his flank exposed. Keep your left arm and leg forward to block a right-handed attack. As he lunges for your throat or face, step forward and sideways by scooting your left leg diagonally across his direction of movement.

## ...BLOCK...

Smack his arm aside using the slap block with your left arm. Hit him just above the elbow. If he is wearing a jacket, grab the sleeve. He'll be deflected by your block, exposing his flank to you.

## ...AND...

Drop your right arm onto his and use the combined force of both your arms to drive him further off course. This negates the danger of him retaliating with his other fist. It's too awkward for him to reach across his body. Lift your right leg. Bring the knee up high.

### ... STOMP.

Side stomp the back of his knee. Drive his leg to the floor. You now have control over his upper and lower body. Pull him further off balance and elbow him in the face with your right arm. If you can master these steps, you will be very difficult to beat.

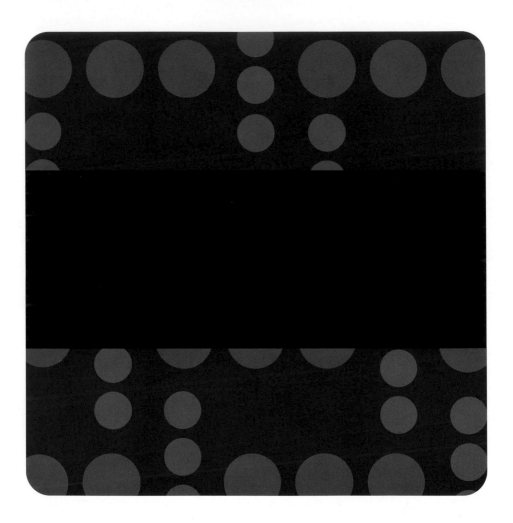

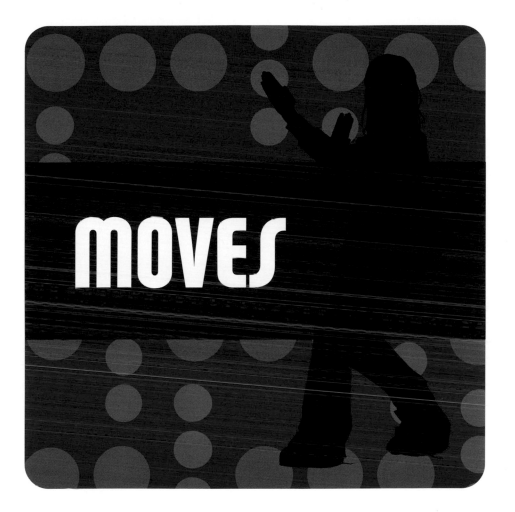

## The Getaway

This man is so angry he seems to want to eat your whole head. He's going for you with both hands. Step in toward him, reach between his arms, and grab his ears hard.

Holding his head like a steering wheel, make a sharp right or left turn. His head will tip in whichever direction you steer it because he wants to keep it attached to his ears.

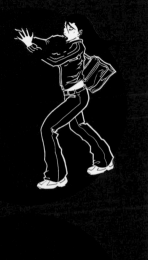

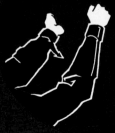

Control his head and you control his balance. Steer him over sideways and kick him in the balls. Let go of his ears when he is thoroughly off balance. Finish him off with a knee strike. If you throw him slightly backward, a kick will work just as well.

He will drop to the floor enveloped in great suffocating waves of pain and self-pity. If the situation is now under control, you can walk away. If not, stomp on his ankle or knee while he is down so he can't chase you if he gets up.

# Back Seat Special

You're sitting on a bus, train, or a park bench. Suddenly, a guy has his arm wrapped around your neck. He tries to drag you away by putting you in a neck lock. He will squeeze hard, but the following counter-attack works even when the lock is on tight. It's also effective when you're standing up.

He's trying to choke you. Reach over his arm as shown. Then chop your arm up into his throat or chin. His head will tip back. Slide your hand up over his face and, for a truly efficient non-slip grip, get your fingers in his eyes and nostrils. Keep his head back at all costs.

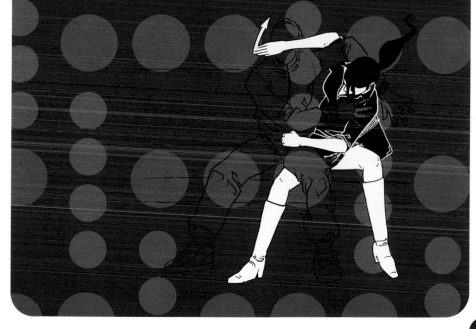

It's now time for your second incapacitating technique of the evening. Punch him where it hurts most. Ignore the garbled pleas for mercy—they are obviously insincere—and hit him again. A couple of good whacks in the groin are enough to soften any man's resolve. Keep his head back.

Stand up and hit him in the throat with a "Y" hand strike. Use the web of skin between your fingers and outstretched thumb to hit his throat. Now find another seat to sit on. This one will be quite a mess.

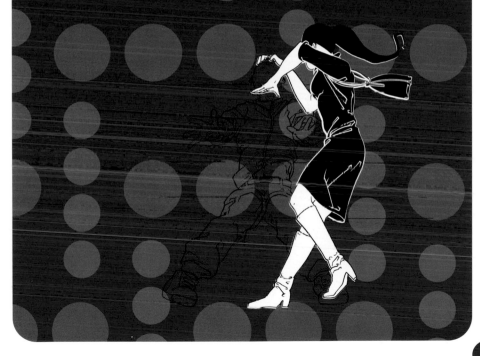

# The Folding Villain

You dozed off on the train. When you wake up, a scary man in a nylon track suit, white leather loafers, and no socks has placed his hand on your thigh. The car is empty apart from one man who suddenly gets interested in his newspaper. You will get no help from him.

Grab the assailant's wrist and place your other hand on his shoulder blade. You can hook your leg around his to increase the amount of control you will have over him later, but the technique works without it. Act fast because he'll be offended that you didn't like him feeling you up.

Pull his wrist up and stretch his arm away in the direction of the arrow. Then lever his shoulder forward and down so that it rotates in the joint and locks. If you've used your leg to trap him, he will possibly have a hyperextended knee at this point.

Stand up. Keep pulling and pushing in the direction of the arrows. Make sure you are balanced, then drop kick his head. Aim for the nose or put your toe in his eye. Then drop him and leave. Try not to start a fight with the loser holding the newspaper.

# Your Butt Is a Weapon

You suddenly are grabbed from behind, and a man tries to drag you away. If he puts his hand over your mouth to stop you from screaming, bite his fingers. Repeatedly stomp on his foot till you get the desired reaction. Grind your heel down his shin. Then slam your elbows into his ribs.

This next move is quite a revelation. Your butt is a weapon! Lift your arms in a rapid arc to snap his grip, and slam your buttocks backward into his gonads. He will double over and lose balance. This technique looks a bit like a silly '60s dance move, but it works.

Stick your arms out like chicken wings, and spin around to deliver a reverse elbow strike to the head or neck. If you've bumped him back out of range, move in quickly to finish him off with a kick to the knee or groin. Just pick your targets until he's writhing on the floor in pain, no longer a threat.

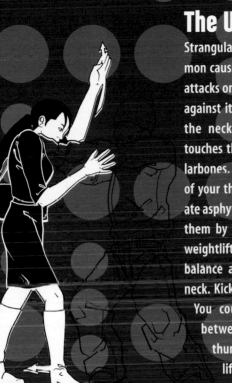

# The Wind Mill

Strangulation is one of the most common causes of death or injury during attacks on women, so learn to defend against it. When he's holding you by the neck, drop your chin until it touches the notch between your collarbones. This hides the weakest part of your throat and prevents immediate asphyxiation. Grab his elbows. Lift them by pushing up as if you were weightlifting. You will throw him off balance and take pressure off your neck. Kick him straight in the groin. You could also work your arms between his and stick your thumbs in his eyes. Or you could lift your arm as indicated and pull back the opposite leg.

Sweep your arm down in a hacking arc, using the low windshield-wiper block to effectively break the stranglehold and trap his arms. Pin his arms against his body with your blocking arm. You could now reverse elbow strike him with your left arm. Just follow the arrow.

Execute a palm strike to the underside of the nose or chin to drive his head back and knock him off balance. You can also gouge his eyes.

If he's still in range, grab both his shoulders and yank him forward for a knee strike to the groin. Pull him hard. The whiplash will disorient him. If he's farther away, kick him. Either way, he will fall like a dead tree.

# Barroom Brawler

Contrary to popular belief, you should not swing chairs in a fight. It's too slow, and if the chair breaks you will be deprived of a useful weapon. It makes much more sense to grip the chair as illustrated and jab at your opponent with the legs. Furthermore, by rotating your hands in a steering wheel motion similar to that described in The Getaway (page 68), you add a whole new dimension to your line of defense.

Here, the chair becomes an effective deterrent and can be used to fend off even the most savage and determined assailants. Why do you think it's so popular with lion-tamers?

You know those awkward little tables that four of you try to squeeze around for your after-work drink? They're supported by a single trunk that splays out to form feet. They look great but are completely unstable if leaned on. Well, there is a better use for this foolish item of furniture. Should a situation deteriorate beyond the point of no return and you need to make a speedy escape (or help a friend), tip over the nearest table, pick it up by the stem or feet, and hold it before you like the shield of Spartacus. Use it to deflect hurled bottles, chairs, glasses, and aggressive customers.

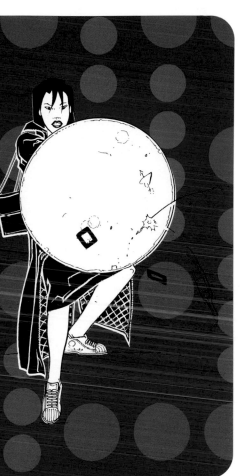

Long banquet tables are common in bars nowadays, and they will probably have bench seating. Either the table or bench can be utilized as a weapon. You might find them a bit on the heavy side, so why not share the load with a friend? With women on either end, sweep the crowd aside. Be determined and maintain a steady course for the nearest exit to escape the attacking thugs. Long tables and benches act like the squeegees used by those annoying guys who try to clean your car windshield at traffic lights, except the gray scummy residue you're left with at the end is made of people, not soap. The chair and table techniques are also extremely effective defenses should you ever have to fight off an intruder in your own home.

# Barry the Bar Bruiser

Barry the Bar Bruiser: the man with no self-restraint or shame. The drunker he is, the worse he gets. As you stand at the bar minding your own business, Barry sidles up and drapes his arm around your shoulders. He mumbles something dull and inconsequential in your ear. Then he oversteps the line and grabs your boob.

Drape your arm over his shoulder by looping it under his armpit and then coming over the top. Simultaneously, reach across with your free hand and grab your own wrist.

Sharply pull with your free hand and push with your other arm to smash his nose on the bar. Give Barry's head a couple of good whacks on the Formica top. You now have him in a shoulder lock. His struggles only aggravate the locked shoulder. All you have to do is lean away from any attempted attack.

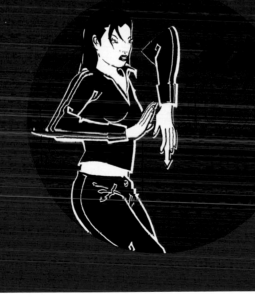

If properly executed, this technique is so quick that there is hardly time for his booze-addled brain to figure out how he got himself into such a ludicrous predicament.

Finishing options:

① Douse him with his own beer.

② Call security and have him ejected from the premises.

# Beat an Attacker with Your Cell Phone

Grab your mobile phone as shown. It's irrelevant which way as long as there is a good portion protruding. Even better—if your phone has an antenna that juts out the top, use it; it has more penetrating power than the base. At moments like this, it's you against him, so you can't afford to be tentative in your movements. Just keep thrashing away, hitting him with the phone till you get the desired result. He needn't be lying down for you to use this technique. Areas to aim for are the eyes, forehead, nose, cheekbones, temples, mouth, ears, throat, and the base of the neck around the collar-bones. With enough force, anywhere you hit him will hurt. Pens, keys, pencils, combs, bits of old wood, your high heels—all can be used in the same effective way.

# Antiknife Technique

There is only one antiknife technique where you're guaranteed not to get slashed or stabbed to death. As mentioned on page 9, it's called TA-RA, which stands for "Turn Around and Run Away."

Avoid a fight at all costs. Turn tail. There is nothing wrong with being terrified. Use the fear constructively to run like the wind. Scream and shout. Make it plain to the whole street that you don't want your attacker near you. Sometimes this will be enough to scare him off. If not, throw things at him to create opportunities for escape. Use anything at hand. Be creative, and always aim at his face. Try to temporarily blind him while you get out of there.

Pieces of clothing wrapped around your arm make good shields until you can get away. So do garbage can lids or even the whole garbage can. You can also keep him at bay with your feet. Use the kicks described earlier to attack him from the waist down. Remember, however: even a trained martial artist is wary of a knife, so if you want to learn how to deal with this situation, don't learn it from a book. Sign up for self-defense classes.

# Antiknife Side Step

If suddenly confronted by a knife attacker, you can use your key fist as defense (see illustration on page 48). As with the side step 45 maneuver (page 62), step toward your attacker at a 45-degree angle. Cut across him as he lunges, making him overshoot the mark and leaving his flank exposed for attack. Lead with your left arm and left leg to block a right-handed attack, and vice versa. As the man lunges for your throat, chest, or face, step forward and to the side by scooting your left leg diagonally across his direction of movement.

Smack his arm aside using the slap block (page 27) with your left arm. Aim to hit him just above the elbow. If he's wearing a jacket, grab the sleeve and shove his arm aside. This forces his arm across his body, spinning him around and exposing his flank.

When you've pushed his arm down, across, and out of the way, gouge his face open with your keys. This is no time for squeamish sensibilities—if you don't cut him, he'll probably hurt you.

# The Clothes Line

Begin the maneuver in the same position as the antiknife technique (page 97). Use the same side step and slap block to avoid his attack. Then place your other leg behind his in order to trip him. Notice that the rear hand is lifted high.

Place your tripping leg behind and between his and slice your arm down. Shove his arm aside with your blocking hand and chop down with the free hand.

His arm will drop when struck. Slide your arm straight up and clothes-line him in the neck with your forearm. If he gags and sticks his tongue out, hit his chin. Hook backward with a small leg movement to enhance his fall. He'll be down for the count, and you can get out of there.

# Twist and Stomp

This move can be useful in a number of ways. If you've been grabbed by the throat, lost your balance, and fallen to the floor, or you are already on the floor and the man is trying to get on top of you and pin you down, use this move.

Drop your chin until it touches the notch between your collarbones. Push your arms between his and grab his head with both hands. Dig your nails in, work your thumbs into his eyes, and drag his head forward to bite his nose. Plant your foot on his thigh. Push out with your foot, hard. His leg will be forced back straight out behind him and he will lose his balance.

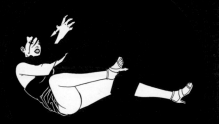

Steer his head sideways, away from the kicking leg. In this case, the right arm rotates up and the left arm down, twisting his neck at an unbearable angle. He will go with it because you have your thumbs in his eyes. Jerk your shoulders off the floor in the direction his head is twisting. Thrust him in the direction he is falling with your kicking leg and push him off.

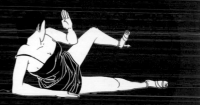

When he lands, he won't be able to see you because you had your thumbs in his eyes and chewed his nose. If this didn't discourage him and he still looks active, stomp on his crown jewels with your stiletto heel. Get up and run.

# Buckaroo

A fat drunk guy is trying to brain you with a beer bottle. Grab his arms by the inside crook of each elbow. Then lift your knee and slam it into his coccyx. He will jerk forward off balance. Buck your hips up and to one side, then steer him off and to one side.

Steer him in the same direction you bucked him in. Lift your shoulders off the ground and roll him away to the side. Finish him with a side stomp kick (page 38). Aim for something soft (not his head). Keep stomping till he looks queasy, then get up and run away.

# The Ear Spanker

A man is holding your friend down, choking her, banging her head on the floor, or trying to assault her. Whatever the case, she doesn't want him there. You rush to your friend's aid.

Reach over his head and grab his face. It's important to get a point of reference in a struggle like this—there's always a lot of movement, confusion, and noise.

Go for the lips, nostrils, and eyes. Claw his head backward and administer a good spanking to the ear. Cup the striking hand as if you were holding water. This creates a hollow palm, which, when slammed over the ear, creates a seal and fills the brute's head with thunderous noise and blinding light. Keep hitting him until he falls. Get your friend up and run.

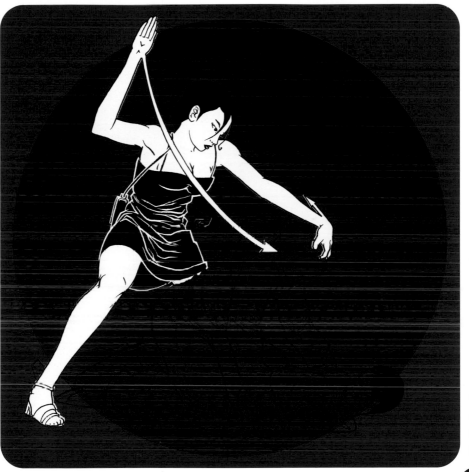

## Stomp Kick Sneak Attack

You're out with your friends when a fight erupts. A man grabs your friend from behind and starts to choke or drag her away. Run up behind him and grab his shoulders, then stomp on the back of his knee. Use the side stomp (page 38) or the cross-stomp kick (page 40). Pull back and down with both arms and thrust your foot toward the ground at the angle indicated.

The thug will tip backward. Reach around and grab his throat. Drag him further off balance until he is falling over. Pull him down far enough to get him in range of your finishing move—in this case, a downward elbow strike. Jump clear as he hits the deck. Your friend wIll be eternally grateful. Now would be a good time to ask her for any money she owes you.

At the end of the day, you are a nice, civilized person being confronted by someone who is not. Ultimately, I want you to walk (or run) away from any attack safe and sound. But if you have to defend yourself, be sure to scream, shout, kick, scratch, bite, and spit. Vomit on him, if it comes to that. Fight back, and make him regret his decision to pick you as a target. If your fighting is precise, measured, and accurate, he will stand little chance. You will walk away unharmed and a little wiser. That's good enough for me.

# Index

antiknife sidestep, 97–99
antiknife technique, 94–99
attitude, 12
awareness and antisurveillance, 13

back seat special, 70–73
barroom brawler, 88
Barry the Bar Bruiser, 89–92
beat an attacker with your cell phone, 93
blocks, 22–27
    circling inner, 26
    circling outer, 25
    double-handed, 23
    inside to the side of the head, 22
    lifting, 24
    low windshield-wiper, 27
    slap, 27
buckaroo, 104–105

cell phones, as weapons, 45, 93
center line, the, 18

chairs, as weapons, 85–86
clothes line, the, 100–101
coins, as weapons, 45
combs, as weapons, 45

destroying movie myths, 35

ear spanker, the, 106–107

folding villain, the, 74–77

getaway, the, 68–69
give him the elbow, 52–54
give him the finger, 57
guard positions, 17

handbag kung fu, 45
high heels, as weapons, 46–49

keep it simple, simple is effective, 8
keys, as weapons, 48
kicks, 36–41
    cross-stomp, 40
    dog lifts its leg, the, 39

kicks *(continued)*
    front groin, 36–37
    give him the boot, 41
    side stomp, 38
KISSIE, 8

lipstick, as a weapon, 45

mascara, as a weapon, 45
muscle memory, 14

objects, as weapons
    banquet tables, 88
    beer, 92
    benches, 88
    cell phones, 45, 93
    chairs, 85–86
    coins, 45
    combs, 45
    handbag, 45
    high heels, 46–49
    keys, 45, 48
    lipstick, 45
    mascara, 45
    tables, 87

palm strikes, 42–44
    give him five, 44
    hook palm, 43
practice, 14

side step 45, 62
stance, 15
stiletto kung fu, 46–49
stomp kick sneak attack, 108–109

TA–RA, 9
tables, as weapons, 87, 88
targets, 20–21
techniques, 53–65
tools, 30–31
transitional phases, 13
turn around and run away, 9
twist and stomp, 102–103

weak points of an attacker, 20–21
wind mill, the, 81–84